MAKEUP ARTIST
EYE CHARTS

FROM THE BEAUTY STUDIO COLLECTION

colorista BOOKS

www.coloristabooks.com

MAKEUP ARTIST EYE CHARTS
Copyright © 2017 by Colorista Books

All rights reserved. No part of this book may be reproduced in any form or by any electronic or mechanical means including information storage and retrieval systems – except in the case of brief quotations in articles or reviews – without the permission in writing from its publisher, Colorista Books.

All brand names and product names used in this book are trademarks, registered trademarks, or trade names of their respective holders. We are not associated with any product or vendor in this book.

Cover designer: Gina Reyna
Interior layout: Gina Reyna
Illustrator: Holly Christie (@avecholly)

OWN THE ENTIRE

Beauty Studio Collection

For the makeup artist & beauty lover in you!

FACE | EYES | LIPS | BROWS | BRIDAL | SCULPT + SHAPE

See the entire collection at:
COLORISTABOOKS.COM

Contents

USER GUIDE

Getting Started	6
Pro Tips + Tricks	7
Drawing Eyelashes	9
Drawing Eyebrows	12

PRACTICE CHARTS

Brow Charts	15
All Eyes	19
Almond Eyes	21
Asian Eyes	23
Round Eyes	25
Hooded Eyes	27
Upturned Eyes	29
Downturned Eyes	31

EYE CHARTS

Almond Eyes	33
Asian Eyes	45
Round Eyes	57
Hooded Eyes	69
Upturned Eyes	81
Downturned Eyes	93

138 total eye charts - 23 of each shape. Half face charts come with & without brows so you have the option of drawing your own.

BONUS MAKEUP CHARTS

Lip Charts	105	Male Face Charts	117
Brow Charts	111	Bridal Face Charts	121
Original Face Charts	113	Sculpt + Shape Chart	125

ABOUT THE CREATOR 129

Sample makeup charts from other books in the Beauty Studio Collection!

GETTING STARTED

This book contains practice charts, makeup charts and bonus makeup charts for hours of coloring fun! Follow the User Guide to discover tips, techniques, and how-to's to customize your makeup looks like a pro!

Color & customize your makeup charts with colored pencils, markers, crayons, even real makeup! Makeup charts include product/color logs so you can easily keep track of what you use for each look.

Build your skills with practice charts

COLORING WITH MAKEUP

Dry makeup formulas such as powder eyeshadow, blush, bronzer & flesh-tone face powders blend easily on paper. An advantage of powder, is that it can be removed with an eraser. White erasers are recommended over colored ones as they are less likely to stain.

You may find cream & liquid products diffcult to use as they tend to apply blotchy & can leave oil stains. However, is possible to use these types of products if you apply them in thin layers. See **'Pro Tips + Tricks'**, to learn more about cream & liquid application techniques.

ABOUT PAPER TEXTURE

Paper texture or "tooth" is about how the surface of paper feels. The more tooth paper has, the rougher it will feel because it has lots of tiny bumps & grooves. Makeup face charts within this book are printed on paper with little tooth, giving it a fairly smooth texture. Now, depending on your choice of coloring material(s), you may find that some products adhere better than others.

Keep track of products + colors

If certain products/colors aren't applying as vibrant as you would like, consider adding some tooth to the paper. An easy ways to do this is with texture hairspray (aerosol) - simply mist the surface of the paper with a thin layer and let dry.

Another way to add tooth is with clear gesso paste.* Apply a thin even layer with a wide synthetic paint brush and let dry. Rinse brush with water immediately after use. If paper feels too gritty, gently smooth surface with fine sandpaper.

* Clear Gesso by Liquitex, Artist's Acrylic or Dina Wakley is recommended.

HOW TO BUILD A PORTFOLIO

Create your own makeup portfolio to showcase your skills & looks. All you'll need are scissors, 8.5" x 11" (3-ring) binder & clear protective sleeves. Cut along dashed line to remove makeup chart from book & put in protective sleeve.

Use binder tab dividers to categorize & organize looks by makeup styles (day, night, bridal, dramatic, smokey eyes, etc..) and/or makeup looks for various skintones (fair, light, med, tan, dark).

Alternatively, you can leave makeup charts in book and use sticky note tab labels to catergorize and organize.

MAKEUP APPLICATION TOOLS

When it comes to applying makeup on a chart, you'll find that smaller brushes offer more control over placement & blending. The most useful eye brushes include:

Dome Blender
Powder, blush, bronzer, contour and highlight

Flat Shader
Eyeshadow and contour

Pointed Pencil
Lip color and defining eyes

Angled Liner
Eyeliner, lip liner & defining brows

user guide
PRO TIPS + TRICKS

Adding Skincolor

• Add any shade of skin color to a makeup chart with flesh tone face powder and a dome blender brush.

• For smooth even results, pick up powder with brush then dab on back of hand to distribute powder evenly into the bristles. Use light circular motions to color in "skin". Repeat until you have reached your desired shade.

• Avoid whites of eyes as you shade in skin. If any makeup gets onto the eyes, use a white eraser to remove it. Alternatively, you can mask the eyeballs before you color the skin with removable tape or a thin coat of clear nail polish.

Powder Makeup

For smooth application - pick up powder with brush & dab on back of hand to distribute evenly into the bristles. Use small circular motions when blending color on paper. Repeat until you reach desired shade.

Cream + Liquid Makeup

The key to achieving the best results with cream & liquid makeup is to apply in thin layers.

HOW TO APPLY CREAMS + LIQUIDS:

1. Put a little makeup on back of your hand.

2. Pick up makeup with dome blender brush.

3. Use dabbing & circular motions on back of hand to evenly distribute makeup into the bristles.

4. Apply color on paper with gentle swiping & circular motions.

5. Repeat steps 1-4 until you reach desired shade.

Eye Enhancements

• For a realistic eye color effect mix blue, green or orange eyeshadow with a bit of brown and/or grey eyeshadow. Fill in eye color with a pointed pencil brush.

• Add a coat of clear shiny nail polish over eye color for a natural glossy effect.

• Keep eraser handy to remove makeup that gets on whites of eyes.

Eyeliner Tips

• Apply a clear nail polish (matte or glossy top coat) over creamy eye pencils or liquid eyeliner to seal & keep from smudging.

• Substitute creamy eyeliner with products that dry and won't smudge. China Markers (by Dixon or Sharpie) make a great substitute for eye pencils. Fine-point permanent markers (by Sharpie) or ink (used with dip pen) can give you the look of rich liquid liner.

• Create the look of white eyeliner with liquid white-out corrector (look for it in a fine-point pen by BIC or Sharpie).

• Dark eyeshadow can be used in place of pencil & liquid eyeliners. For sharp crisp lines, apply with an angled liner brush. For a soft & smokey effect, line eyes with a pointed pencil brush.

user guide
PRO TIPS + TRICKS

Sparkle Effect

Glitter is a fun & easy way to add a touch of glitz & glam to your makeup looks.

HOW TO APPLY GLITTER:

1. Use brush or finger to spread an even layer of clear school or craft glue onto makeup chart (applying glue with tool will provide more even coverage).
2. Pour glitter over glue.
3. Hold makeup chart upright and tap to get rid of excess glitter. Be sure to lay paper under makeup chart to catch extra glitter.

Metallic Pigments

Highly-reflective metallic finishes are a great way to add a dimension and shine to makeup charts. For best results, use metallic pigments in powder form (eyeshadow, loose pigment, etc...). For application of liquid metallic makeup see tip on **'Cream + Liquid Makeup'**.

HOW TO APPLY METALLIC PIGMENTS:

1. Pick up powder on flat shader brush.
2. Lightly mist with water until slightly damp.
3. Distribute powder & water into the bristles by gently dabbing on the back of your hand.
4. Apply on paper with dabbing/pressing motions & let dry.
5. Use dry dome blender brush & metallic powder to blur any hard lines (use small circular motions along edges to create a seamless blend).

Cleaning Brushes

Using the same brush for multiple applications can easily lead to "muddy" colors. A simple way to avoid this is with a quick "dry cleaning" in between applications to remove color residue left on bristles. Simply wipe your brush on a damp baby wipe (or damp paper towel with a little baby shampoo lather). Then wipe bristles on a dry paper towel to remove excess moisture.

Adding Highlights

Highlights give face charts a pro look by adding dimension. Highlights can be easily achieved with the 'Reverse Highlighting Technique' - simply add color to makeup chart then use an eraser to remove color where you want highlights to be.

Lip Color

• Substitute creamy lip products with powder eyeshadow or colored pencils.

• Real lipgloss is not recommended for makeup charts as it can easily smear. A great substitute for lip gloss is shiny clear nail polish. Apply a coat of clear shiny nail polish over lips for glossy effect.

• Create your own custom tinted "lipgloss" by mixing clear nail polish & powder eyeshadow.

• To create a tinted gloss in a shade similar to real lips, mix clear nail polish with peachy-mauve eyeshadow or blush. Add matte white eyeshadow to lighten and make more opaque.

HOW TO MAKE TINTED LIPGLOSS:

1. Cut a square piece of foil (about 4 x 4 inches). Gently push a finger into the center of foil to create a bowl.

2. Pour clear nail polish in bowl until 1/4 - 1/2 full.

3. Scrap a little bit of eyeshadow into bowl using needle or toothpick.

4. Mix powder & polish well with applicator brush.

5. Test color on white piece of scrap paper. Keep adding eyeshadow & testing until you reach desired shade. If color is too dark, add more clear polish or white eyeshadow.

6. Apply color to lips immediatley.
Clean applicator brush with nail polish remover before dipping back into polish bottle.

Set and Seal

Protect & preserve completed face charts from moisture, fading and smearing with an 'artist fixative' or 'paper protectant' spray. You will need a well-ventilated area when using these types of products - please follow directions carefully!
*Krylon Preserve It Matte' is recommended.

how-to tutorial
DRAWING EYELASHES

A full set of lashes is a fab way to customize your makeup charts. When it comes to drawing lashes, you'll want to use a drawing tool that's opaque, adheres to paper over makeup & is fine enough to create delicate lash "hairs" with.

Liquid eyeliner, sharpie markers & dark color pencils are common drawing tools but can sometimes be challenging to work with because they either aren't fine enough to draw fine lash strokes with or don't show up very good over eyeshadow.

A far better option, although a little untraditional, is ink & a dip pen. India/Sumi ink is thin yet opaque & permanent when dry. When used together with a dip pen & a fine-nib, you can create thick to thin hair-like strokes with smooth precision. Speedball offers inexpensive ink & dip pen sets (Sketching or Mapping Project Set is recommended).

In this tutorial you will learn how to draw 4 styles of lashes. Each style varies in density giving your a range of looks from light to ultra full & dramatic. But before we jump into drawing full sets of lashes, it's helpful to begin with the basics. 'Drawing Lashes 101' will guide you on drawing individual "lash hairs".

Eyelash Styles

Natural   Wispy

Glamour   Bombshell

DRAWING LASHES 101

WHAT YOU NEED ☐ Drawing tool ☐ Scrap paper ☐ Eye practice chart

STEP 1: PREP DRAWING TOOL

Pencil user: Sharpen pencil so that you can create fine strokes (lines) that mimic natural lash hairs. Keep sharpener handy as point can quickly become dull when drawing.

Dip pen + ink user: Dip nib into ink just past the eye. Scribble on scrap paper to remove excess ink.

Please note: Dried up ink on nibs can be difficult to remove & block ink flow. After every drawing session, it's recommended to clean nibs with window cleaner & an old soft toothbrush. Dry thoroughly with cloth or paper towel to prevent from rusting.

STEP 2: PRACTICE STROKE

A stroke is a line that reduces in thickness towards one end. Real eyelashes resemble curved tapered strokes. To create tapered strokes, press down drawing tool with some pressure begin reducing pressure as you draw a small curved line. On a scrap piece of paper, practice single strokes & clusters of 2-3 strokes (of varying lengths).

STEP 3: PRACTICE STROKE DIRECTION

Open Eye: Starting at inner part of eye draw short strokes (in the same direction as the letter "C") until you reach the iris. At the iris begin drawing strokes the direction as a backwards letter "C". Increase length & tilt of strokes as you move towards outer corner. For bottom lashes, mirror top lashes using shorter strokes.

Closed Eye: Starting at inner part of eye draw short strokes (in the same direction as a backwards letter "C"). Increase length & tilt of stroke as you move along eye towards outer corner.

how-to tutorial
DRAWING EYELASHES

DRAWING LASH STYLES WHAT YOU NEED ☐ Drawing tool ☐ Eye or face chart

Note: Lash strokes were drawn above the eye to provide you with a clear view of the strokes drawn on the lashline.

HOW TO DRAW
Natural Lash Style

1. Draw 1st set of lashes for open & closed eye.

2. Add a few single lashes between gaps.

3. Continue adding single lashes & a few clusters to add fullness. For the most natural look do not fill in all gaps - you should be able to see the eyelid through the lashes.

4. Draw bottom lashes on open eye (optional).

HOW TO DRAW
Wispy Lash Style

1. Draw 1st set of lashes for open & closed eye (draw mostly clusters of varying lengths).

2. Add a few single lashes & clusters of varying lengths between gaps.

3. Continue adding single lashes & clusters. For natural results do not fill in all gaps - you should be able to see the some of the eyelid through the lashes.

4. Draw bottom lashes on open eye (optional).

how-to tutorial
DRAWING EYELASHES

HOW TO DRAW
Bombshell Lash Style

1. Draw 1st set of lashes for open & closed eye. Draw short, med and long clusters. Start with shortest ones near inner corner, med towards center and longest near outer corner.

2. Add a few single lashes and clusters of varying lengths between gaps.

3. Continue adding single lashes & clusters of varying lengths. For the most natural look fill in most gaps (but not all) to create the illusion of fullness.

4. Draw bottom lashes on open eye (optional).

HOW TO DRAW
Glamour Lash Style

1. Draw 1st set of lashes for open & closed eye draw mainly thick clusters of varying lengths).

2. Add a single lashes & clusters of varying lengths between gaps.

3. Continue adding single lashes & clusters of varing lengths to increase density (fill in the majority of gaps-you shouldn't be able to see much of the eyelid through the lashes).

4. Draw bottom lashes on open eye (optional).

how-to tutorial
DRAWING EYEBROWS

Similarly to lashes, brows can play a important role in a makeup look. Although are many styles of brows, they can be simplified down to 5 shapes of varying thickness: Straight, Round, Soft angle, Sharp Angle & S-shape.

When it comes to drawing brows on paper, you'll want to choose a drawing tool that allows you to create hair-like strokes with precision. You'll find that lead/colored pencils or thin markers work best for brows as they offer a fine point, come in natural brow shades and won't smudge like creamy eye/brow pencils do.

It's important to note that drawing brows involves erasing, so you may want to consider applying eye or face after brows application (this will eliminate having to reapply makeup that you accidently removed/erased).

To get started, follow 'Brow Drawing Basics' to become familiar with drawing realistic brow hairs. When you are ready to draw your own custom brows, follow 'How to Draw Brows from Scratch'.

BROW DRAWING BASICS

WHAT YOU NEED
- ☐ Pencil (lead or colored) ☐ Sharpener ☐ Scrap paper
- ☐ Eye or brow chart

STEP 1: PREP TOOL

Sharpen pencil so that you can create fine strokes (lines) that mimic natural brow hairs. Keep sharpener handy as point can quickly become dull when drawing.

STEP 2: PRACTICE STROKES

A stroke is a line that reduces in thickness towards on end. Real brow hairs resemble curved tapered strokes. Brow hairs generally grow straight up at the inner part of the brow and then begin to tilt outwards.

On a scrap peice of paper, practice single strokes of varying lengths. To create a tapered stroke, press pencil down with some pressure - begin reducing pressure as you draw a small curved line.

STEP 3: PRACTICE STROKE DIRECTION

Fill in pre-outlined brow with hair strokes:

LEFT BROW: Start at inner part of brow, draw a few vertical strokes then start tilting strokes outwards to the LEFT - when you reach the highest point of the arch shorten length of strokes.

RIGHT BROW: Start at inner part of brow, draw a few vertical strokes then start tilting strokes outwards to the RIGHT - when you reach the highest point of the arch shorten length of strokes.

how-to tutorial
DRAWING EYEBROWS

DRAWING BROWS FROM SCRATCH

WHAT YOU NEED
☐ Ruler ☐ Pencil ☐ Eraser ☐ Pencil brush ☐ Brow powder
☐ Colored pencil (in brow shade of choice)

PART ONE
Mapping Brows

Follow the 3 point method to determine where a brow starts, highest point of arch & where it ends. Use a ruler & pencil to lightly mark points. When mapping brows, consider the space between the lid & brows. Higher placement offers more space for eyeshadow but can also create a permanently surprised look.

A. Beginning of brow aligns with center of nostril.

B. Highest point of arch aligns with edge of nostril and center of iris (on closed eye measure to approximately center of eye).

C. End of brow aligns with edge of nostril & the outer corner of eye.

Example of low, medium & high brow placement

PART TWO
Outline + Fill

1. After mapping brows, use pencil to lightly sketch an outline of the brow shape. Keep eraser handy to make corrections as needed.

2. With a colored pencil, fill in shape with hairlike strokes. Start at beginning with a few vertical strokes then fill in rest of shape with tilted strokes.*

3. Lightly erase pencil marks & brow outline.

4. Fill in sparse areas with brow powder & pencil brush.

5. Use colored pencil to redefine strokes. Add more strokes of various lengths in sparse areas for extra dimension & definition.

6. Use eraser lightly around edges of brows to clean up any smudges and further define shape. Touch up and/or add more hairstrokes in sparse areas (optional).

 PRO TIPS *If you have trouble sketching brow shape outline freehand, try using a brow stencil.*

Steps 4-6 can be used to further enhance pre-drawn or pre-outlined brows that have been filled in with brow hairs.

BROW PRACTICE CHARTS

Use templates to fill in pre-outlined brow shapes

NOTES

Straight

Round

Soft Angle

Sharp Angle

S-shape

BLANK BROW PRACTICE CHARTS

Use templates to draw brows from scratch by mapping, outlining shape and filliing in.

NOTES

EYE PRACTICE CHARTS

Use templates to design looks and practice application techniques.

All Shapes Eye Open

Almond — Asian (monolid) — Round

Hooded — Upturned — Downturned

NOTES _____

All Shapes Eye Closed

Almond — Asian (monolid) — Round

Hooded — Upturned — Downturned

NOTES _____

EYE PRACTICE CHARTS

Use templates to design looks and practice application techniques.

Almond Eye Open

NOTES _____

Almond Eye Closed

NOTES _____

EYE PRACTICE CHARTS

Use templates to design looks and practice application techniques.

Asian (monolid) Eye Open

NOTES _____
_____

Asian (monolid) Eye Closed

NOTES _____
_____

23

EYE PRACTICE CHARTS

Use templates to design looks and practice application techniques.

Round Eye Open

NOTES _____

_____

Round Eye Closed

NOTES _____

_____

EYE PRACTICE CHARTS

Use templates to design looks and practice application techniques.

Hooded Eye Open

NOTES _____

Hooded Eye Closed

NOTES _____

EYE PRACTICE CHARTS

Use templates to design looks and practice application techniques.

Upturned Eye Open

Upturned Eye Closed

NOTES _____

NOTES _____

EYE PRACTICE CHARTS

Use templates to design looks and practice application techniques.

Downturned Eye Open

NOTES _____

Downturned Eye Closed

NOTES _____

makeup eye charts
Almond Shape

makeup eye charts

LOOK NAME _____
EYE SHAPE _Almond_____
BROWS _____
LINER _____
EYE SHADOW _____
_____
LASHES _____

LOOK NAME _____
EYE SHAPE _Almond_____
BROWS _____
LINER _____
EYE SHADOW _____
_____
LASHES _____

LOOK NAME _____
EYE SHAPE _Almond_____
BROWS _____
LINER _____
EYE SHADOW _____
_____
LASHES _____

LOOK NAME _____
EYE SHAPE _Almond_____
BROWS _____
LINER _____
EYE SHADOW _____
_____
LASHES _____

BRUSHES + TOOLS

_____

_____

_____

_____

NOTES

_____

_____

_____

_____

BRUSHES + TOOLS

_____

_____

_____

_____

NOTES

_____

_____

_____

_____

BRUSHES + TOOLS

_____

_____

_____

_____

NOTES

_____

_____

_____

_____

BRUSHES + TOOLS

_____

_____

_____

_____

NOTES

_____

_____

_____

_____

makeup eye charts

LOOK NAME _____
EYE SHAPE _Almond_____
BROWS _____
LINER _____
EYE SHADOW _____
_____
LASHES _____

LOOK NAME _____
EYE SHAPE _Almond_____
BROWS _____
LINER _____
EYE SHADOW _____
_____
LASHES _____

LOOK NAME _____
EYE SHAPE _Almond_____
BROWS _____
LINER _____
EYE SHADOW _____
_____
LASHES _____

LOOK NAME _____
EYE SHAPE _Almond_____
BROWS _____
LINER _____
EYE SHADOW _____
_____
LASHES _____

BRUSHES + TOOLS

_____
_____
_____
_____

....

NOTES

_____
_____
_____
_____

....

BRUSHES + TOOLS

_____
_____
_____
_____

....

NOTES

_____
_____
_____
_____

....

BRUSHES + TOOLS

_____
_____
_____
_____

....

NOTES

_____
_____
_____
_____

....

BRUSHES + TOOLS

_____
_____
_____
_____

NOTES

_____
_____
_____
_____

makeup eye chart

LOOK NAME _____
EYE SHAPE _Almond_____
BROWS _____
EYESHADOW _____
_____

MASCARA _____
LASHES _____
NOTES _____
CLIENT NAME _____
MAKEUP ARTIST _____

makeup eye chart

LOOK NAME _____
EYE SHAPE _Almond_____
BROWS _____
EYESHADOW _____
_____

MASCARA _____
LASHES _____
NOTES _____
CLIENT NAME _____
MAKEUP ARTIST _____

BRUSHES + TOOLS

_____
_____
_____
_____

NOTES

_____
_____
_____
_____

BRUSHES + TOOLS

_____
_____
_____
_____

NOTES

_____
_____
_____
_____

makeup eye chart

LOOK NAME _____
EYE SHAPE __Almond_____
BROWS _____
EYESHADOW _____
_____

MASCARA _____
LASHES _____
NOTES _____
CLIENT NAME _____
MAKEUP ARTIST _____

makeup eye chart

LOOK NAME _____
EYE SHAPE __Almond_____
BROWS _____
EYESHADOW _____
_____

MASCARA _____
LASHES _____
NOTES _____
CLIENT NAME _____
MAKEUP ARTIST _____

BRUSHES + TOOLS

_____
_____
_____
_____

NOTES

_____
_____
_____
_____

BRUSHES + TOOLS

_____
_____
_____
_____

NOTES

_____
_____
_____
_____

makeup eye chart

LOOK NAME _____
EYE SHAPE _Almond_____
BROWS _____
EYESHADOW _____
_____

MASCARA _____
LASHES _____
NOTES _____
CLIENT NAME _____
MAKEUP ARTIST _____

makeup eye chart

LOOK NAME _____
EYE SHAPE _Almond_____
BROWS _____
EYESHADOW _____
_____

MASCARA _____
LASHES _____
NOTES _____
CLIENT NAME _____
MAKEUP ARTIST _____

BRUSHES + TOOLS

NOTES

BRUSHES + TOOLS

NOTES

makeup eye charts
Asian (monolid) Shape

makeup eye charts

LOOK NAME _____
EYE SHAPE _Asian (monolid)_____
BROWS _____
LINER _____
EYE SHADOW _____
_____
LASHES _____

LOOK NAME _____
EYE SHAPE _Asian (monolid)_____
BROWS _____
LINER _____
EYE SHADOW _____
_____
LASHES _____

LOOK NAME _____
EYE SHAPE _Asian (monolid)_____
BROWS _____
LINER _____
EYE SHADOW _____
_____
LASHES _____

LOOK NAME _____
EYE SHAPE _Asian (monolid)_____
BROWS _____
LINER _____
EYE SHADOW _____
_____
LASHES _____

BRUSHES + TOOLS

_____
_____
_____
_____

NOTES

_____
_____
_____
_____

BRUSHES + TOOLS

_____
_____
_____
_____

NOTES

_____
_____
_____
_____

BRUSHES + TOOLS

_____
_____
_____
_____

NOTES

_____
_____
_____
_____

BRUSHES + TOOLS

_____
_____
_____
_____

NOTES

_____
_____
_____
_____

makeup eye charts

LOOK NAME _____
EYE SHAPE Asian (monolid) _____
BROWS _____
LINER _____
EYE SHADOW _____
_____
LASHES _____

LOOK NAME _____
EYE SHAPE Asian (monolid) _____
BROWS _____
LINER _____
EYE SHADOW _____
_____
LASHES _____

LOOK NAME _____
EYE SHAPE Asian (monolid) _____
BROWS _____
LINER _____
EYE SHADOW _____
_____
LASHES _____

LOOK NAME _____
EYE SHAPE Asian (monolid) _____
BROWS _____
LINER _____
EYE SHADOW _____
_____
LASHES _____

BRUSHES + TOOLS

_____

_____

_____

_____

NOTES

_____

_____

_____

_____

....

BRUSHES + TOOLS

_____

_____

_____

_____

NOTES

_____

_____

_____

_____

....

BRUSHES + TOOLS

_____

_____

_____

_____

NOTES

_____

_____

_____

_____

....

BRUSHES + TOOLS

_____

_____

_____

_____

NOTES

_____

_____

_____

_____

makeup eye chart

LOOK NAME _____
EYE SHAPE Asian (monolid) _____
BROWS _____
EYESHADOW _____
_____

MASCARA _____
LASHES _____
NOTES _____
CLIENT NAME _____
MAKEUP ARTIST _____

makeup eye chart

LOOK NAME _____
EYE SHAPE Asian (monolid) _____
BROWS _____
EYESHADOW _____
_____

MASCARA _____
LASHES _____
NOTES _____
CLIENT NAME _____
MAKEUP ARTIST _____

BRUSHES + TOOLS

NOTES

BRUSHES + TOOLS

NOTES

makeup eye chart

LOOK NAME _____
EYE SHAPE _Asian (monolid)_____
BROWS _____
EYESHADOW _____
_____

MASCARA _____
LASHES _____
NOTES _____
CLIENT NAME _____
MAKEUP ARTIST _____

makeup eye chart

LOOK NAME _____
EYE SHAPE _Asian (monolid)_____
BROWS _____
EYESHADOW _____
_____

MASCARA _____
LASHES _____
NOTES _____
CLIENT NAME _____
MAKEUP ARTIST _____

BRUSHES + TOOLS

_____
_____
_____
_____

NOTES

_____
_____
_____
_____

BRUSHES + TOOLS

_____
_____
_____
_____

NOTES

_____
_____
_____
_____

makeup eye chart

LOOK NAME _____
EYE SHAPE __Asian (monolid)_____
BROWS _____
EYESHADOW _____
_____

MASCARA _____
LASHES _____
NOTES _____
CLIENT NAME _____
MAKEUP ARTIST _____

makeup eye chart

LOOK NAME _____
EYE SHAPE __Asian (monolid)_____
BROWS _____
EYESHADOW _____
_____

MASCARA _____
LASHES _____
NOTES _____
CLIENT NAME _____
MAKEUP ARTIST _____

BRUSHES + TOOLS

NOTES

BRUSHES + TOOLS

NOTES

makeup eye charts
Round Shape

makeup eye charts

LOOK NAME _____
EYE SHAPE _Round_____
BROWS _____
LINER _____
EYE SHADOW _____
_____
LASHES _____

LOOK NAME _____
EYE SHAPE _Round_____
BROWS _____
LINER _____
EYE SHADOW _____
_____
LASHES _____

LOOK NAME _____
EYE SHAPE _Round_____
BROWS _____
LINER _____
EYE SHADOW _____
_____
LASHES _____

LOOK NAME _____
EYE SHAPE _Round_____
BROWS _____
LINER _____
EYE SHADOW _____
_____
LASHES _____

BRUSHES + TOOLS

NOTES

BRUSHES + TOOLS

NOTES

BRUSHES + TOOLS

NOTES

BRUSHES + TOOLS

NOTES

makeup eye charts

LOOK NAME _____
EYE SHAPE Round _____
BROWS _____
LINER _____
EYE SHADOW _____
_____
LASHES _____

LOOK NAME _____
EYE SHAPE Round _____
BROWS _____
LINER _____
EYE SHADOW _____
_____
LASHES _____

LOOK NAME _____
EYE SHAPE Round _____
BROWS _____
LINER _____
EYE SHADOW _____
_____
LASHES _____

LOOK NAME _____
EYE SHAPE Round _____
BROWS _____
LINER _____
EYE SHADOW _____
_____
LASHES _____

BRUSHES + TOOLS

_____

_____

_____

_____

....

BRUSHES + TOOLS

_____

_____

_____

_____

....

BRUSHES + TOOLS

_____

_____

_____

_____

....

BRUSHES + TOOLS

_____

_____

_____

_____

NOTES

_____

_____

_____

_____

NOTES

_____

_____

_____

_____

NOTES

_____

_____

_____

_____

NOTES

_____

_____

_____

_____

makeup eye chart

LOOK NAME _____
EYE SHAPE _Round_ _____
BROWS _____
EYESHADOW _____
_____

MASCARA _____
LASHES _____
NOTES _____
CLIENT NAME _____
MAKEUP ARTIST _____

makeup eye chart

LOOK NAME _____
EYE SHAPE _Round_ _____
BROWS _____
EYESHADOW _____
_____

MASCARA _____
LASHES _____
NOTES _____
CLIENT NAME _____
MAKEUP ARTIST _____

BRUSHES + TOOLS

_____
_____
_____
_____

NOTES

_____
_____
_____
_____

BRUSHES + TOOLS

_____
_____
_____
_____

NOTES

_____
_____
_____
_____

makeup eye chart

LOOK NAME _____
EYE SHAPE __Round_____
BROWS _____
EYESHADOW_____
_____

MASCARA _____
LASHES _____
NOTES _____
CLIENT NAME _____
MAKEUP ARTIST _____

makeup eye chart

LOOK NAME _____
EYE SHAPE __Round_____
BROWS _____
EYESHADOW_____
_____

MASCARA _____
LASHES _____
NOTES _____
CLIENT NAME _____
MAKEUP ARTIST _____

BRUSHES + TOOLS

_____
_____
_____
_____

NOTES

_____
_____
_____
_____

BRUSHES + TOOLS

_____
_____
_____
_____

NOTES

_____
_____
_____
_____

makeup eye chart

LOOK NAME _____
EYE SHAPE _Round_ _____
BROWS _____
EYESHADOW _____
_____

MASCARA _____
LASHES _____
NOTES _____
CLIENT NAME _____
MAKEUP ARTIST _____

makeup eye chart

LOOK NAME _____
EYE SHAPE _Round_ _____
BROWS _____
EYESHADOW _____
_____

MASCARA _____
LASHES _____
NOTES _____
CLIENT NAME _____
MAKEUP ARTIST _____

BRUSHES + TOOLS

_____
_____
_____
_____

NOTES

_____
_____
_____
_____

BRUSHES + TOOLS

_____
_____
_____
_____

NOTES

_____
_____
_____
_____

makeup eye charts
Hooded Shape

makeup eye charts

LOOK NAME _____
EYE SHAPE _Hooded_____
BROWS _____
LINER _____
EYE SHADOW _____
_____
LASHES _____

LOOK NAME _____
EYE SHAPE _Hooded_____
BROWS _____
LINER _____
EYE SHADOW _____
_____
LASHES _____

LOOK NAME _____
EYE SHAPE _Hooded_____
BROWS _____
LINER _____
EYE SHADOW _____
_____
LASHES _____

LOOK NAME _____
EYE SHAPE _Hooded_____
BROWS _____
LINER _____
EYE SHADOW _____
_____
LASHES _____

71

BRUSHES + TOOLS

_____
_____
_____
_____

NOTES

_____
_____
_____
_____

....

BRUSHES + TOOLS

_____
_____
_____
_____

NOTES

_____
_____
_____
_____

....

BRUSHES + TOOLS

_____
_____
_____
_____

NOTES

_____
_____
_____
_____

....

BRUSHES + TOOLS

_____
_____
_____
_____

NOTES

_____
_____
_____
_____

makeup eye charts

LOOK NAME _____
EYE SHAPE Hooded _____
BROWS _____
LINER _____
EYE SHADOW _____
_____
LASHES _____

LOOK NAME _____
EYE SHAPE Hooded _____
BROWS _____
LINER _____
EYE SHADOW _____
_____
LASHES _____

LOOK NAME _____
EYE SHAPE Hooded _____
BROWS _____
LINER _____
EYE SHADOW _____
_____
LASHES _____

LOOK NAME _____
EYE SHAPE Hooded _____
BROWS _____
LINER _____
EYE SHADOW _____
_____
LASHES _____

BRUSHES + TOOLS

_____
_____
_____
_____

....

NOTES

_____
_____
_____
_____

BRUSHES + TOOLS

_____
_____
_____
_____

....

NOTES

_____
_____
_____
_____

BRUSHES + TOOLS

_____
_____
_____
_____

....

NOTES

_____
_____
_____
_____

BRUSHES + TOOLS

_____
_____
_____
_____

NOTES

_____
_____
_____
_____

makeup eye chart

LOOK NAME _____
EYE SHAPE Hooded _____
BROWS _____
EYESHADOW _____
_____

MASCARA _____
LASHES _____
NOTES _____
CLIENT NAME _____
MAKEUP ARTIST _____

makeup eye chart

LOOK NAME _____
EYE SHAPE Hooded _____
BROWS _____
EYESHADOW _____
_____

MASCARA _____
LASHES _____
NOTES _____
CLIENT NAME _____
MAKEUP ARTIST _____

BRUSHES + TOOLS

_____
_____
_____
_____

NOTES

_____
_____
_____
_____

BRUSHES + TOOLS

_____
_____
_____
_____

NOTES

_____
_____
_____
_____

makeup eye chart

LOOK NAME _____
EYE SHAPE Hooded _____
BROWS _____
EYESHADOW _____
_____

MASCARA _____
LASHES _____
NOTES _____
CLIENT NAME _____
MAKEUP ARTIST _____

makeup eye chart

LOOK NAME _____
EYE SHAPE Hooded _____
BROWS _____
EYESHADOW _____
_____

MASCARA _____
LASHES _____
NOTES _____
CLIENT NAME _____
MAKEUP ARTIST _____

BRUSHES + TOOLS

_____
_____
_____
_____

NOTES

_____
_____
_____
_____

BRUSHES + TOOLS

_____
_____
_____
_____

NOTES

_____
_____
_____
_____

makeup eye chart

LOOK NAME _____
EYE SHAPE Hooded _____
BROWS _____
EYESHADOW _____
_____

MASCARA _____
LASHES _____
NOTES _____
CLIENT NAME _____
MAKEUP ARTIST _____

makeup eye chart

LOOK NAME _____
EYE SHAPE Hooded _____
BROWS _____
EYESHADOW _____
_____

MASCARA _____
LASHES _____
NOTES _____
CLIENT NAME _____
MAKEUP ARTIST _____

BRUSHES + TOOLS

_____
_____
_____
_____

....

NOTES

_____
_____
_____
_____

BRUSHES + TOOLS

_____
_____
_____
_____

NOTES

_____
_____
_____
_____

makeup eye charts
Upturned Shape

makeup eye charts

LOOK NAME _____
EYE SHAPE _Upturned_____
BROWS _____
LINER _____
EYE SHADOW _____
_____
LASHES _____

LOOK NAME _____
EYE SHAPE _Upturned_____
BROWS _____
LINER _____
EYE SHADOW _____
_____
LASHES _____

LOOK NAME _____
EYE SHAPE _Upturned_____
BROWS _____
LINER _____
EYE SHADOW _____
_____
LASHES _____

LOOK NAME _____
EYE SHAPE _Upturned_____
BROWS _____
LINER _____
EYE SHADOW _____
_____
LASHES _____

BRUSHES + TOOLS

_____

_____

_____

_____

NOTES

_____

_____

_____

_____

BRUSHES + TOOLS

_____

_____

_____

_____

NOTES

_____

_____

_____

_____

BRUSHES + TOOLS

_____

_____

_____

_____

NOTES

_____

_____

_____

_____

BRUSHES + TOOLS

_____

_____

_____

_____

NOTES

_____

_____

_____

_____

makeup eye charts

LOOK NAME _____
EYE SHAPE Upturned _____
BROWS _____
LINER _____
EYE SHADOW _____
_____
LASHES _____

LOOK NAME _____
EYE SHAPE Upturned _____
BROWS _____
LINER _____
EYE SHADOW _____
_____
LASHES _____

LOOK NAME _____
EYE SHAPE Upturned _____
BROWS _____
LINER _____
EYE SHADOW _____
_____
LASHES _____

LOOK NAME _____
EYE SHAPE Upturned _____
BROWS _____
LINER _____
EYE SHADOW _____
_____
LASHES _____

BRUSHES + TOOLS

_____
_____
_____
_____

....

NOTES

_____
_____
_____
_____

BRUSHES + TOOLS

_____
_____
_____
_____

....

NOTES

_____
_____
_____
_____

BRUSHES + TOOLS

_____
_____
_____
_____

....

NOTES

_____
_____
_____
_____

BRUSHES + TOOLS

_____
_____
_____
_____

NOTES

_____
_____
_____
_____

makeup eye chart

LOOK NAME _____
EYE SHAPE _Upturned_ _____
BROWS _____
EYESHADOW _____
_____

MASCARA _____
LASHES _____
NOTES _____
CLIENT NAME _____
MAKEUP ARTIST _____

....

makeup eye chart

LOOK NAME _____
EYE SHAPE _Upturned_ _____
BROWS _____
EYESHADOW _____
_____

MASCARA _____
LASHES _____
NOTES _____
CLIENT NAME _____
MAKEUP ARTIST _____

BRUSHES + TOOLS

_____
_____
_____
_____

NOTES

_____
_____
_____
_____

BRUSHES + TOOLS

_____
_____
_____
_____

NOTES

_____
_____
_____
_____

makeup eye chart

LOOK NAME _____
EYE SHAPE Upturned _____
BROWS _____
EYESHADOW _____
_____

MASCARA _____
LASHES _____
NOTES _____
CLIENT NAME _____
MAKEUP ARTIST _____

makeup eye chart

LOOK NAME _____
EYE SHAPE Upturned _____
BROWS _____
EYESHADOW _____
_____

MASCARA _____
LASHES _____
NOTES _____
CLIENT NAME _____
MAKEUP ARTIST _____

BRUSHES + TOOLS

_____
_____
_____
_____

NOTES

_____
_____
_____
_____

BRUSHES + TOOLS

_____
_____
_____
_____

NOTES

_____
_____
_____
_____

makeup eye chart

LOOK NAME _____
EYE SHAPE _Upturned_ _____
BROWS _____
EYESHADOW _____
_____

MASCARA _____
LASHES _____
NOTES _____
CLIENT NAME _____
MAKEUP ARTIST _____

makeup eye chart

LOOK NAME _____
EYE SHAPE _Upturned_ _____
BROWS _____
EYESHADOW _____
_____

MASCARA _____
LASHES _____
NOTES _____
CLIENT NAME _____
MAKEUP ARTIST _____

BRUSHES + TOOLS

NOTES

BRUSHES + TOOLS

NOTES

makeup eye charts
Downturned Shape

makeup eye charts

LOOK NAME _____
EYE SHAPE _Downturned_____
BROWS _____
LINER _____
EYE SHADOW _____
_____
LASHES _____

LOOK NAME _____
EYE SHAPE _Downturned_____
BROWS _____
LINER _____
EYE SHADOW _____
_____
LASHES _____

LOOK NAME _____
EYE SHAPE _Downturned_____
BROWS _____
LINER _____
EYE SHADOW _____
_____
LASHES _____

LOOK NAME _____
EYE SHAPE _Downturned_____
BROWS _____
LINER _____
EYE SHADOW _____
_____
LASHES _____

BRUSHES + TOOLS

NOTES

BRUSHES + TOOLS

NOTES

BRUSHES + TOOLS

NOTES

BRUSHES + TOOLS

NOTES

makeup eye charts

LOOK NAME _____
EYE SHAPE _Downturned_____
BROWS _____
LINER _____
EYE SHADOW _____
_____
LASHES _____

LOOK NAME _____
EYE SHAPE _Downturned_____
BROWS _____
LINER _____
EYE SHADOW _____
_____
LASHES _____

LOOK NAME _____
EYE SHAPE _Downturned_____
BROWS _____
LINER _____
EYE SHADOW _____
_____
LASHES _____

LOOK NAME _____
EYE SHAPE _Downturned_____
BROWS _____
LINER _____
EYE SHADOW _____
_____
LASHES _____

BRUSHES + TOOLS

_____
_____
_____
_____

....

NOTES

_____
_____
_____
_____

....

BRUSHES + TOOLS

_____
_____
_____
_____

....

NOTES

_____
_____
_____
_____

....

BRUSHES + TOOLS

_____
_____
_____
_____

....

NOTES

_____
_____
_____
_____

....

BRUSHES + TOOLS

_____
_____
_____
_____

NOTES

_____
_____
_____
_____

makeup eye chart

LOOK NAME _____
EYE SHAPE _Downturned_____
BROWS _____
EYESHADOW _____
_____

MASCARA _____
LASHES _____
NOTES _____
CLIENT NAME _____
MAKEUP ARTIST _____

makeup eye chart

LOOK NAME _____
EYE SHAPE _Downturned_____
BROWS _____
EYESHADOW _____
_____

MASCARA _____
LASHES _____
NOTES _____
CLIENT NAME _____
MAKEUP ARTIST _____

BRUSHES + TOOLS

_____
_____
_____
_____

NOTES

_____
_____
_____
_____

BRUSHES + TOOLS

_____
_____
_____
_____

NOTES

_____
_____
_____
_____

makeup eye chart

LOOK NAME _____
EYE SHAPE _Downturned_____
BROWS _____
EYESHADOW _____
_____

MASCARA _____
LASHES _____
NOTES _____
CLIENT NAME _____
MAKEUP ARTIST _____

makeup eye chart

LOOK NAME _____
EYE SHAPE _Downturned_____
BROWS _____
EYESHADOW _____
_____

MASCARA _____
LASHES _____
NOTES _____
CLIENT NAME _____
MAKEUP ARTIST _____

BRUSHES + TOOLS

_____
_____
_____
_____

NOTES

_____
_____
_____
_____

BRUSHES + TOOLS

_____
_____
_____
_____

NOTES

_____
_____
_____
_____

makeup eye chart

LOOK NAME _____
EYE SHAPE Downturned _____
BROWS _____
EYESHADOW _____
_____

MASCARA _____
LASHES _____
NOTES _____
CLIENT NAME _____
MAKEUP ARTIST _____

makeup eye chart

LOOK NAME _____
EYE SHAPE Downturned _____
BROWS _____
EYESHADOW _____
_____

MASCARA _____
LASHES _____
NOTES _____
CLIENT NAME _____
MAKEUP ARTIST _____

BRUSHES + TOOLS

NOTES

BRUSHES + TOOLS

NOTES

makeup lip charts
Full Shape

makeup lip charts

LOOK NAME _____

LIP SHAPE Thin-upper

LINER _____
COLOR _____
GLOSS _____

NOTES _____
_____
_____
_____

LOOK NAME _____

LIP SHAPE Medium

LINER _____
COLOR _____
GLOSS _____

NOTES _____
_____
_____
_____

LOOK NAME _____

LIP SHAPE Full

LINER _____
COLOR _____
GLOSS _____

NOTES _____
_____
_____
_____

BRUSHES + TOOLS

NOTES

BRUSHES + TOOLS

NOTES

BRUSHES + TOOLS

NOTES

makeup lip chart

LOOK NAME _____
LIP SHAPE Full _____
LINER _____
COLOR _____

GLOSS _____
NOTES _____
CLIENT NAME _____
MAKEUP ARTIST _____

makeup lip chart

LOOK NAME _____
LIP SHAPE Full _____
LINER _____
COLOR _____

GLOSS _____
NOTES _____
CLIENT NAME _____
MAKEUP ARTIST _____

BRUSHES + TOOLS

_____

_____

_____

....

NOTES

_____

_____

_____

....

BRUSHES + TOOLS

_____

_____

_____

NOTES

_____

_____

_____

makeup brow charts

NAME _____
BROW SHAPE Straight

NAME _____
BROW SHAPE Round

NAME _____
BROW SHAPE Soft Arch

NAME _____
BROW SHAPE Sharp Arch

NAME _____
BROW SHAPE S-shape

makeup face chart

LOOK NAME

_____

EYES

Brows: _____

Base: _____

Eye shadow: _____

_____

_____

Eyeliner: _____

Mascara: _____

Lashes: _____

FACE

Primer: _____

Concealer: _____

Foundation: _____

Powder: _____

Blush: _____

Bronzer: _____

Contour: _____

Highlight: _____

LIPS

Liner: _____

Gloss: _____

Color: _____

_____

CLIENT NAME

_____

MAKEUP ARTIST

_____

113

BRUSHES + TOOLS

_____
_____
_____
_____
_____

NOTES

_____
_____
_____
_____
_____

makeup face chart

LOOK NAME

_____

EYES

Brows: _____
Base: _____
Eye shadow: _____
_____
_____
Eyeliner: _____
Mascara: _____
Lashes: _____

FACE

Primer: _____
Concealer: _____
Foundation: _____
Powder: _____
Blush: _____
Bronzer: _____
Contour: _____
Highlight: _____

LIPS

Liner: _____
Gloss: _____
Color: _____
_____

CLIENT NAME

_____

MAKEUP ARTIST

_____

BRUSHES + TOOLS

_____
_____
_____
_____
_____

NOTES

_____
_____
_____
_____
_____

makeup face chart

LOOK NAME

_____

EYES

Brows:_____

Base:_____

Eye shadow:_____

_____

_____

Eyeliner:_____

Mascara:_____

Lashes:_____

FACE

Primer:_____

Concealer:_____

Foundation:_____

Powder:_____

Blush:_____

Bronzer:_____

Contour:_____

Highlight:_____

LIPS

Liner:_____

Gloss:_____

Color:_____

_____

CLIENT NAME

_____

MAKEUP ARTIST

_____

BRUSHES + TOOLS

NOTES

makeup face chart

LOOK NAME

_____

EYES

Brows: _____

Base: _____

Eye shadow: _____

_____

_____

Eyeliner: _____

Mascara: _____

Lashes: _____

FACE

Primer: _____

Concealer: _____

Foundation: _____

Powder: _____

Blush: _____

Bronzer: _____

Contour: _____

Highlight: _____

LIPS

Liner: _____

Gloss: _____

Color: _____

_____

CLIENT NAME

_____

MAKEUP ARTIST

_____

119

BRUSHES + TOOLS

NOTES

bridal face chart

LOOK NAME

_____

EYES

Brows: _____
Base: _____
Eye shadow: _____
_____
_____
Eyeliner: _____
Mascara: _____
Lashes: _____

FACE

Primer: _____
Concealer: _____
Foundation: _____
Powder: _____
Blush: _____
Bronzer: _____
Contour: _____
Highlight: _____

LIPS

Liner: _____
Gloss: _____
Color: _____
_____

CLIENT NAME

_____

MAKEUP ARTIST

_____

BRUSHES + TOOLS

NOTES

WEDDING DETAILS

bridal face chart

LOOK NAME
_____

EYES
Brows: _____
Base: _____
Eye shadow: _____
_____
_____
Eyeliner: _____
Mascara: _____
Lashes: _____

FACE
Primer: _____
Concealer: _____
Foundation: _____
Powder: _____
Blush: _____
Bronzer: _____
Contour: _____
Highlight: _____

LIPS
Liner: _____
Gloss: _____
Color: _____
_____

CLIENT NAME
_____

MAKEUP ARTIST
_____

123

BRUSHES + TOOLS

NOTES

WEDDING DETAILS

how-to tutorial
HIGHLIGHT + CONTOUR

Heart Face Shape
HIGHLIGHT + CONTOUR GUIDE

The highlight and contour method for a **Heart** face shape focuses on minimizing the width of the face and rounding out the strong angular structure of the jaw & point of chin.

STEP 1: CONTOUR

Use dome blender brush and contour powder to shade:

Hairline
Under cheekbones (curved line)
Sides of neck (optional)

Define shading along **hairline & under cheekbones** with flat shader brush & contour powder.

Add shading to **sides of nose & under bottom lip** with pencil brush & contour powder. Also add contour along **tip of chin** to soften sharp angles.

STEP 2: HIGHLIGHT + MID-TONE

Highlights are placed on the high points of the face. Use dome blender brush to apply highlight powder to (or leave areas blank if using white of paper as highlight)::

Forehead
Browbone
Inner eye corners
Under eyes
Cheekbones
Bridge of nose
Cupids bow
Center of chin

Apply mid-tone skincolor to blank areas between contour & highlight. Use small circular motions to create a seamless blend.

STEP 3: BLUSH

Balance sharp angle of jaw and point of chin with a curvy shape - similar to that of a kidney bean.

Apply blush with blender brush for added shape and natural flush of color.

sculpt + shape chart

LOOK NAME _____

FACE SHAPE: Heart _____

HIGHLIGHT _____
CONTOUR _____
MID-TONE _____
FACE _____
_____
_____

EYES _____
_____
_____
_____

LIPS _____
_____
_____

BRUSHES + TOOLS

_____

_____

_____

_____

_____

NOTES

_____

_____

_____

_____

_____

About the Creator

Gina M. Reyna, founder and owner of Colorista Books, has been a professional makeup artist since 2009. She is an Empire Beauty School graduate & has attended fine art classes at the Art Institute and the Academy of Art University San Francisco. Her experience as a makeup artist ranges from weddings & special events to editorial-style photography.

When Gina isn't working as a makeup artist, she spends her time creating content for makeup artists and beauty enthusiasts. Her first book, 'How to be a Professional Makeup Artist - A Comprehensive Guide for Beginners', was published in January of 2013. She has since then written 'The Complete Guide to Smokey Eyes' & created The Beauty Studio Collection of makeup charts.

If you have a question or comment for Gina, please send it to: gina@coloristabooks.com

To learn more visit us at:

COLORISTABOOKS.COM

Made in the USA
Las Vegas, NV
01 September 2022